MEDICAL RESEARCH COUNCIL OF THE U.K.

Memorandum No. 45 (superseding War Memorandum No. 7)

Aids to the examination of the peripheral nervous system

D1188393

PENDRAGON HOUSE

**Aids to the examination of
the peripheral nervous system**

© British Crown copyright 1976.
Reprinted by permission of the Controller of
Her Britannic Majesty's Stationery Office.

First published in the U.S.A. in 1978 by
Pendragon House, Inc., 2595 East Bayshore,
Palo Alto, CA 94303.

First American printing by the George Banta
Company, Inc., Menasha, Wisconsin 54952

Production Editor: H. R. Heinz

International Standard Book Number 0 916 988 15 5

Library of Congress Number 78 54120

Price: $3.50

Preface

The Medical Research Council's pamphlet *Aids to the Investigation of Peripheral Nerve Injuries* (War memorandum No. 7, 1941), revised in 1943 and many times reprinted, has become a standard work. This thoroughly revised successor takes account of the extension of knowledge and the changes in practice over the last 30 years. The new title, *Aids to the Examination of the Peripheral Nervous System*, reflects the use made of the pamphlet by students and practitioners, which is much wider than the war-time emphasis on nerve injuries would have indicated.

Earlier editions of this atlas were prepared by the staff of the Department of Surgery, University of Edinburgh. For this revision many alterations have been made in the text and in the captions. Methods of examining certain muscles not mentioned in previous editions are now illustrated, while one or two muscles which are rarely if ever tested in clinical practice have been omitted. Many of the diagrams have been redrawn and new illustrations showing the approximate distribution of dermatomes have been included. All the photographs have been replaced, as the blocks used in the previous two editions were no longer serviceable after so many impressions. Some of the new illustrations and photographs have been prepared in the Institute of Orthopaedics, London, many in the Department of Medical Illustration and Photography, Guy's Hospital (with the help of Dr M. D. O'Brien) and others at the Institute of Neurology, London. Professor J. Joseph of the Department of Anatomy, Guy's Hospital Medical School, has kindly reviewed the text and illustrations and has made many helpful suggestions.

The Council is indebted to Churchill-Livingstone Limited for permission to include Figure 5 from the second edition of *Surgical Disorders of Peripheral Nerves* (1975) by Sir Herbert Seddon.

Figures 1, 2, 6, 7, 10, 11, 21, 23, 29, 30, 31, 32, 34, 35, 37, 40 and 49 have been reproduced with permission from the Institute of Neurology, National Hospital for Nervous Diseases.

Figures 3, 4, 8, 9, 12, 13, 14, 15, 16, 17, 18, 19, 20, 22, 24, 25, 26, 27, 28, 33, 36, 38, 39, 41, 42, 43, 44, 45, 46, 47, 48, 50, 51, 52, 53, 54, 55, 56, 57, 58, 59, 60, 61, 62, 63, 64, 65, 66, 67, 87, 88 and 90 have been reproduced with permission from Guy's Hospital Medical School.

Medical Research Council   1975
20 Park Crescent
London W1N 4AL

Nerve injuries committee 1943

Brigadier G. Riddoch, MD, FRCP (*Chairman*)
Brigadier W. Rowley Bristow, MB, FRCS
Brigadier H. W. B. Cairns, DM, FRCS
E. A. Carmichael, CBE, MB, FRCP
Surgeon Captain M. Critchley, MD, FRCP, RNVR
J. G. Greenfield, MD, FRCP
Professor J. R. Learmonth, CBE, ChM, FRCSE
Professor H. Platt, MD, FRCS
Professor H. J. Seddon, DM, FRCS
Air Commodore C. P. Symonds, MD, FRCP
J. Z. Young, MA
F. J. C. Herrald, MB, MRCPE (*Secretary*)

Revision subcommittee, 1972-1975

Sir Herbert Seddon, CMG, DM, FRCS (*Chairman until October 1973*)
Professor J. N. Walton, TD, MD, DSc, FRCP (*Chairman from October 1973*)
Professor R. W. Gilliatt, DM, FRCP
M. J. F. McArdle, MB, FRCP
Professor P. K. Thomas, DSc, MD, FRCP
R. G. Willison, DM, FRCPE

Contents

Aids to the examination of the peripheral nervous system

Introduction

This atlas is intended as a guide to the examination of patients with lesions of peripheral nerves and nerve roots.

These examinations should, if possible, be conducted in a quiet room where patient and examiner will be free from distraction. For both motor and sensory testing it is important that the patient should first be warm. The nature and object of the tests should be explained to the patient so that his interest and cooperation are secured. If either shows signs of fatigue the session should be discontinued and resumed later.

Motor testing

A muscle may act as a *prime mover*, as a *fixator*, as an *antagonist*, or as a *synergist*. Thus, flexor carpi ulnaris acts as a *prime mover* when it flexes and adducts the wrist; as a *fixator* when it immobilizes the pisiform bone during contraction of the abductor digiti minimi; as an *antagonist* when it resists extension of the wrist; and as a *synergist* when the digits, but not the wrists, are extended.

As far as possible the action of each muscle should be observed separately and a note made of those in which power has been retained as well as of those that are weak or paralyzed. It is usual to examine the power of a muscle in relation to the movement of a single joint. It has long been customary to use a 0 to 5 scale for recording muscle power, but it is now generally recognized that subdivision of grade 4 may be helpful.

0 No contraction
1 Flicker or trace of contraction
2 Active movement, with gravity eliminated
3 Active movement against gravity
4 Active movement against gravity and resistance
5 Normal power

Grades 4—,4 and 4+, may be used to indicate movement against slight, moderate and strong resistance respectively.

The models employed in this work were not chosen because they showed unusual muscular development; but the ease with which the contraction of muscles is identified varies with the build of the patient, and it is essential that the examiner should both look for and endeavor to feel the contraction of an accessible muscle and/or the movement of its tendon. In most of the illustrations the optimum point for palpation has been marked.

Muscles have been arranged in the order of the origin of their motor supply from nerve trunks, which is convenient in many examinations. Usually only one method of testing each muscle is shown but, where necessary, multiple illustrations have been included if a muscle has more than one important action. The examiner should apply the tests as they are illustrated, because the techniques shown will eliminate many of the traps for the inexperienced provided by "trick" movements. It should be noted that each of the methods used tests, as a rule, the action of muscles at a single joint.

The usual nerve supply to each muscle is stated in the captions, and the spinal segments from which it is derived, the more important of the latter being printed in heavy type. Tables showing limb muscles arranged according to their supply by individual nerve roots and peripheral nerves are to be found on pages (62-63).

Sensory testing

The patient is first asked to outline the area of sensory abnormality; this can be a useful guide to the detailed examination. Light touch should be tested by touches with something soft such as cotton wool, working from the insensitive towards the sensitive area. If the area of sensory abnormality is hypersensitive the direction is reversed. The area delineated is marked by a continuous line. For testing superficial pain a sharp pin is best and again — unless there is apparent hypersensitivity (hyperpathia) — the stimuli are applied first to the analgesic area, working outwards. The area is outlined by a series of dots. The timing of the stimuli should be irregular so that the patient does not know when to expect the next touch or pinprick.

It may also be important to test two-point discrimination on the fingers, joint position sense and, on occasion, deep pressure sense.

The area of skin supplied by any one nerve or nerve root varies from patient to patient, as exemplified by the median (Fig. 75) and ulnar (Fig. 76) nerves. The areas shown in the diagrams are the usual ones.

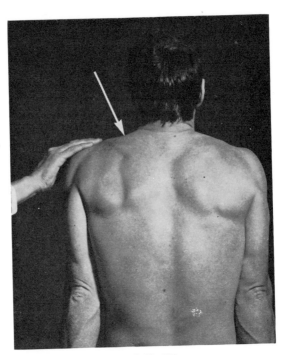

Fig. 1 TRAPEZIUS (Spinal accessory nerve and C3, C4)
The patient is elevating the shoulder against resistance. *Arrow:* the thick upper part of the muscle can be seen and felt.

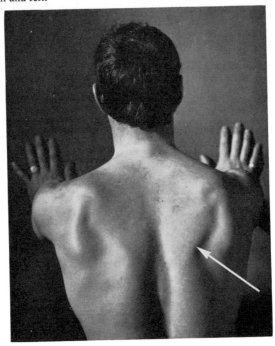

Fig. 2 TRAPEZIUS (Spinal accessory nerve and C3, C4)
The patient is pushing the palms of the hands hard against a wall with the elbows fully extended. *Arrow:* the lower fibres of trapezius can be seen and felt.

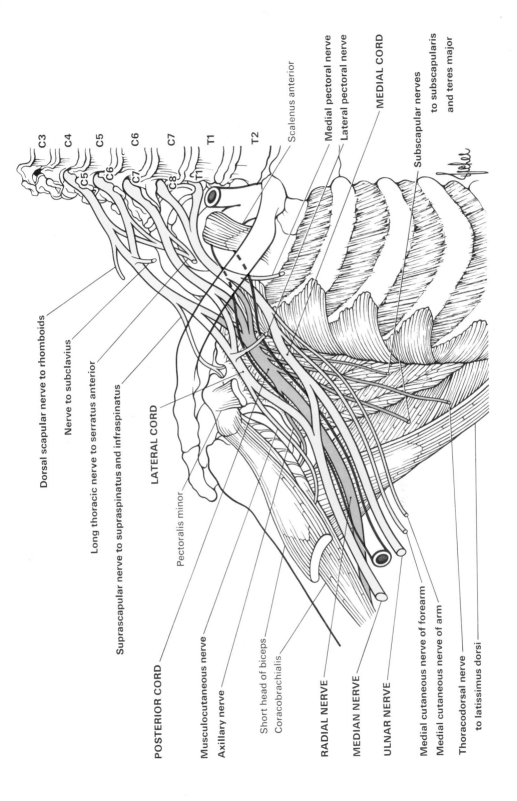

Dorsal scapular nerve to rhomboids

Nerve to subclavius

Long thoracic nerve to serratus anterior

Suprascapular nerve to supraspinatus and infraspinatus

LATERAL CORD

Pectoralis minor

POSTERIOR CORD

Musculocutaneous nerve

Axillary nerve

Short head of biceps

Coracobrachialis

RADIAL NERVE

MEDIAN NERVE

ULNAR NERVE

Medial cutaneous nerve of forearm

Medial cutaneous nerve of arm

Thoracodorsal nerve to latissimus dorsi

C3
C4
C5
C6
C7
T1
T2

C5
C6
C7
C8
T1

Scalenus anterior

Medial pectoral nerve

Lateral pectoral nerve

MEDIAL CORD

Subscapular nerves to subscapularis and teres major

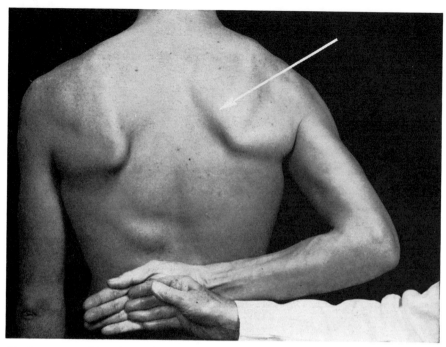

Fig. 4 RHOMBOIDS (Dorsal scapular nerve; C4, C5)
The patient is pressing the palm of his hand backwards against the examiner's hand. *Arrow:* the muscle bellies can be felt and sometimes seen.

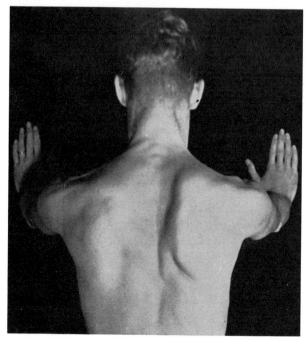

Fig. 5 SERRATUS ANTERIOR (Long thoracic nerve; C5, C6, C7)
The patient is pushing against a wall as in Fig. 2. The right serratus anterior is paralyzed and there is winging of the scapula.

10

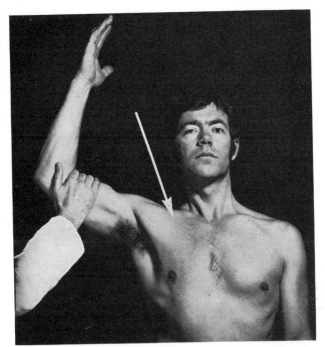

Fig. 6 PECTORALIS MAJOR: CLAVICULAR HEAD (Lateral pectoral nerve; **C5**, C6)
The upper arm is above the horizontal and the patient is pushing forward against the examiner's
hand. *Arrow:* the clavicular head of pectoralis major can be seen and felt.

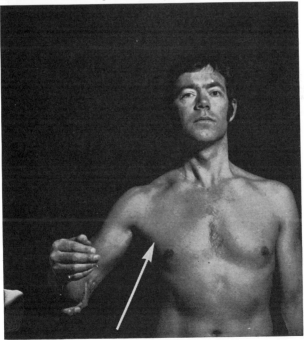

Fig. 7 PECTORALIS MAJOR: STERNOCOSTAL HEAD (Lateral and medial pectoral nerves; C6, **C7**, C8)
The patient is adducting the upper arm against resistance. *Arrow:* the sterno-costal head can
be seen and felt.

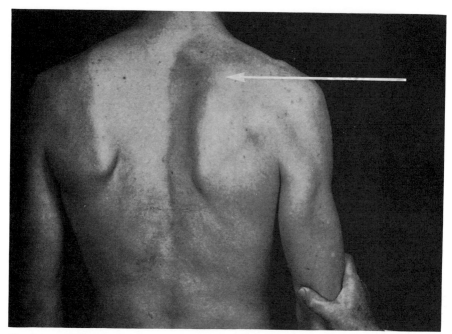

Fig. 8 SUPRASPINATUS (Suprascapular nerve; **C5,** C6)
The patient is abducting the upper arm against resistance. *Arrow:* the muscle belly can be felt and sometimes seen.

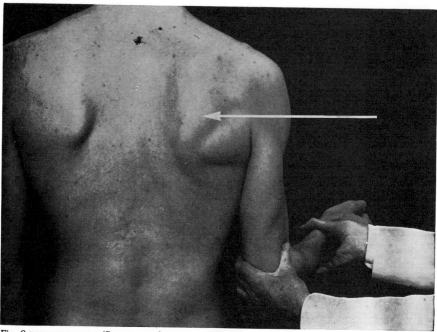

Fig. 9 INFRASPINATUS (Suprascapular nerve; **C5,** C6)
The patient is externally rotating the upper arm at the shoulder against resistance. The examiner's right hand is resisting the movement and supporting the forearm with the elbow at a right angle; his left hand is supporting the elbow and preventing abduction of the arm. *Arrow:* the muscle belly can be seen and felt.

12

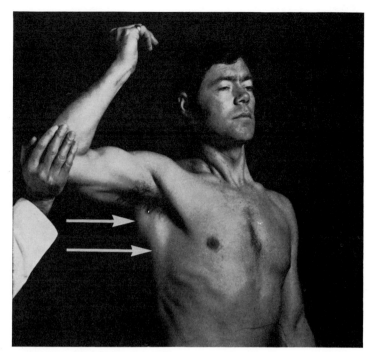

Fig. 10 LATISSIMUS DORSI (Thoracodorsal nerve; C6, **C7,** C8)
The upper arm is horizontal and the patient is adducting it against resistance. *Lower arrow:* the muscle belly can be seen and felt. The upper arrow points to teres major.

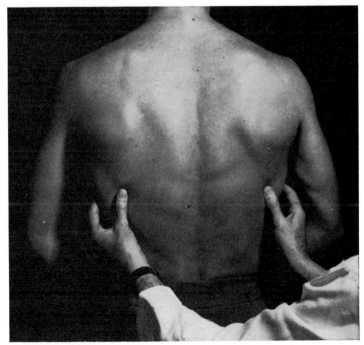

Fig. 11 LATISSIMUS DORSI (Thoracodorsal nerve; C6, **C7,** C8)
The muscle bellies can be felt to contract when the patient coughs.

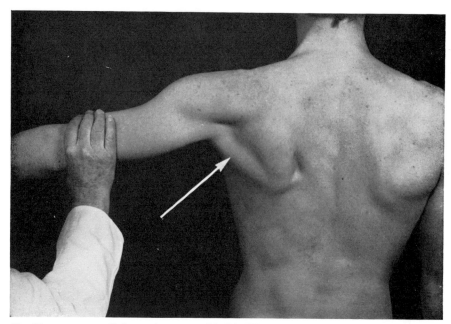

Fig. 12 TERES MAJOR (Subscapular nerve; C5, C6, C7)
The patient is adducting the elevated upper arm against resistance. *Arrow:* the muscle belly can
be seen and felt.

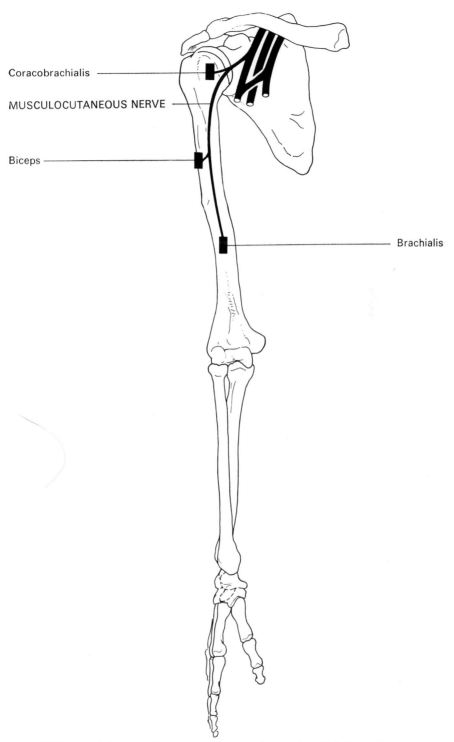

Coracobrachialis

MUSCULOCUTANEOUS NERVE

Biceps

Brachialis

Fig. 13 Diagram of the musculocutaneous nerve and the muscles which it supplies.
(Modified from Pitres and Testut (1925) *Les neufs en Schemas,* Doin, Paris)

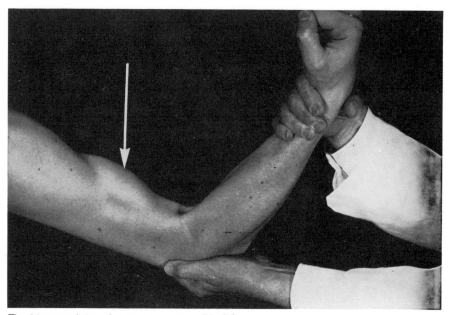

Fig. 14 BICEPS (Musculocutaneous nerve; C5, C6)
The patient is flexing the supinated forearm against resistance. *Arrow:* the muscle belly can be seen and felt.

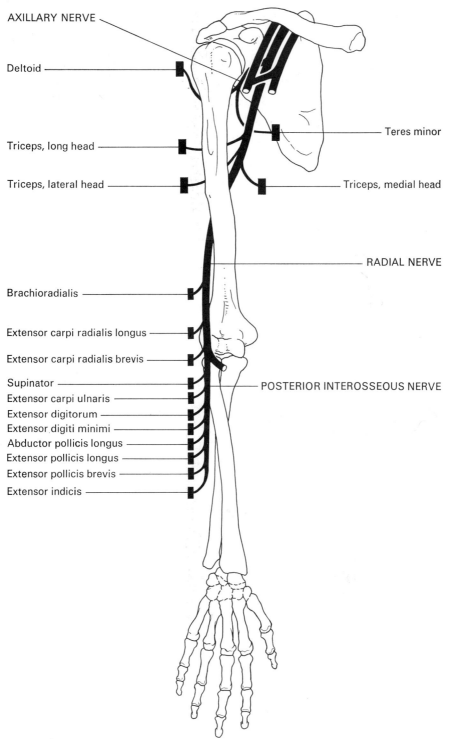

AXILLARY NERVE

Deltoid

Teres minor

Triceps, long head

Triceps, lateral head

Triceps, medial head

RADIAL NERVE

Brachioradialis

Extensor carpi radialis longus

Extensor carpi radialis brevis

Supinator

POSTERIOR INTEROSSEOUS NERVE

Extensor carpi ulnaris

Extensor digitorum

Extensor digiti minimi

Abductor pollicis longus

Extensor pollicis longus

Extensor pollicis brevis

Extensor indicis

Fig. 15 Diagram of the axillary and radial nerves and the muscles which they supply.
(Modified from Pitres and Testut)

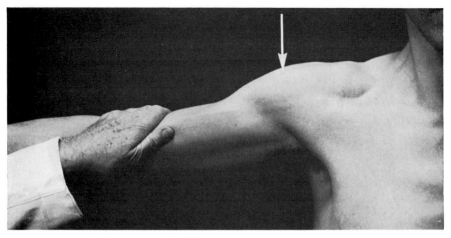

Fig. 16 DELTOID (Axillary nerve; **C5,** C6)
The patient is abducting the upper arm against resistance. *Arrow:* the anterior and middle fibers of the muscle can be seen and felt.

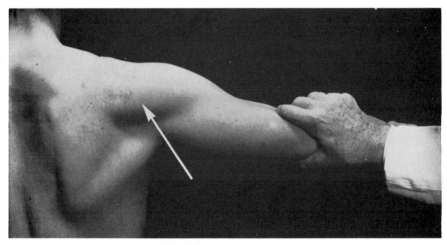

Fig. 17 DELTOID (Axillary nerve: **C5,** C6)
The patient is retracting the abducted upper arm against resistance. *Arrow:* the posterior fibers of deltoid can be seen and felt.

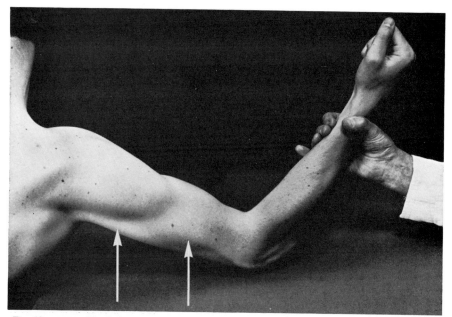

Fig. 18 TRICEPS (Radial nerve; C6, **C7**, C8)
The patient is extending the forearm at the elbow against resistance. The elbow is supported on a table. *Arrows:* the long and lateral heads of the muscle can be seen and felt.

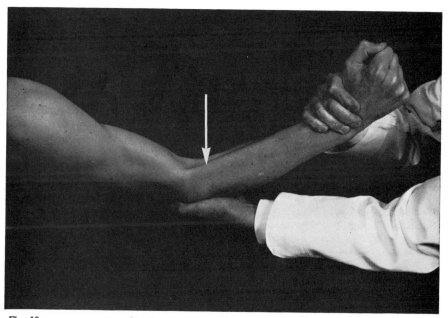

Fig. 19 BRACHIORADIALIS (Radial nerve; C5, **C6**)
The patient is flexing the forearm against resistance with the forearm midway between pronation and supination. *Arrow:* the muscle belly can be seen and felt.

19

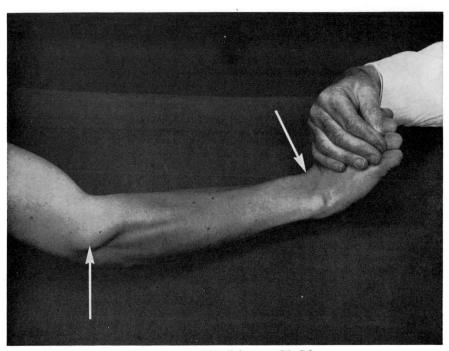

Fig. 20 EXTENSOR CARPI RADIALIS LONGUS (Radial nerve; C5, **C6**)
The patient is extending and abducting the hand at the wrist against resistance. *Arrows:* the muscle belly and tendon can be felt and usually seen.

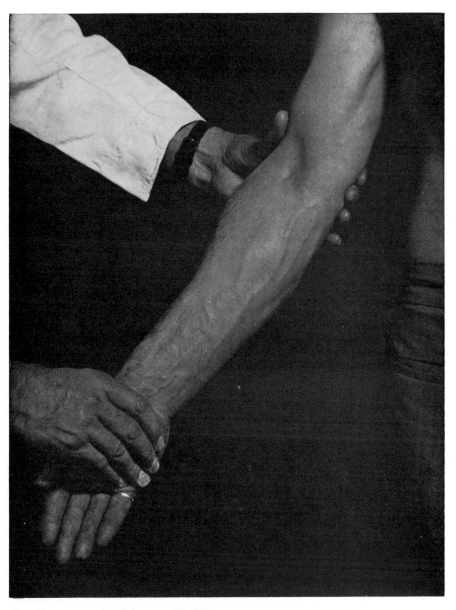

Fig. 21 SUPINATOR (Radial nerve: C6, C7)
The patient is supinating the forearm against resistance with the forearm extended at the elbow.

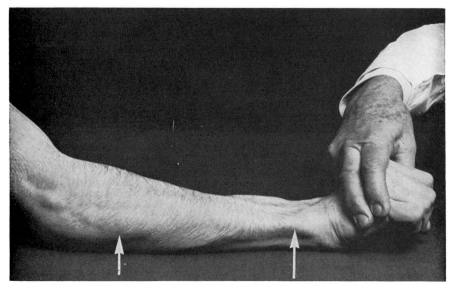

Fig. 22 EXTENSOR CARPI ULNARIS (Posterior interosseous nerve: **C7,** C8)
The patient is extending and adducting the hand at the wrist against resistance. *Arrows:* the muscle belly and the tendon can be seen and felt.

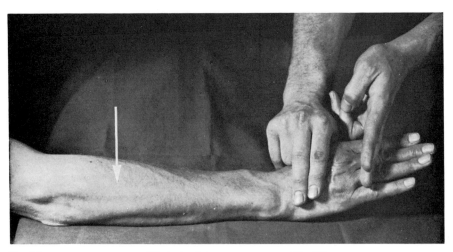

Fig. 23 EXTENSOR DIGITORUM (Posterior interosseous nerve; **C7,** C8)
The patient's hand is firmly supported by the examiner's right hand. Extension at the meta-carpophalangeal joints is maintained against the resistance of the fingers of the examiner's left hand. *Arrow:* the muscle belly can be seen and felt.

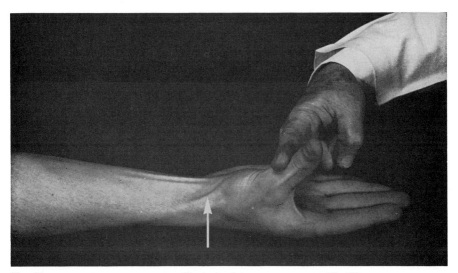

Fig. 24 ABDUCTOR POLLICIS LONGUS (Posterior interosseous nerve; **C7**, C8)
The patient is abducting the thumb at the carpo-metacarpal joint in a plane at right angles to the palm. *Arrow:* the tendon can be seen and felt anterior and closely adjacent to the tendon of extensor pollicis brevis (**cf.** Fig. 26).

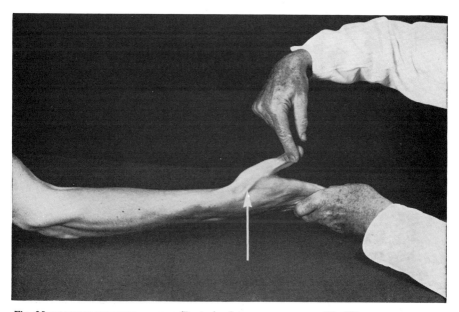

Fig. 25 EXTENSOR POLLICIS LONGUS (Posterior interosseous nerve; **C7**, C8)
The patient is extending the thumb at the interphalangeal joint against resistance. *Arrow:* the tendon can be seen and felt.

23

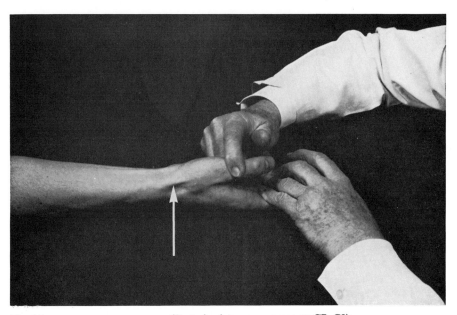

Fig. 26 EXTENSOR POLLICIS BREVIS (Posterior interosseous nerve; **C7,** C8)
The patient is extending the thumb at the metacarpophalangeal joint against resistance. *Arrow:* the tendon can be seen and felt (**cf.** Fig. 24).

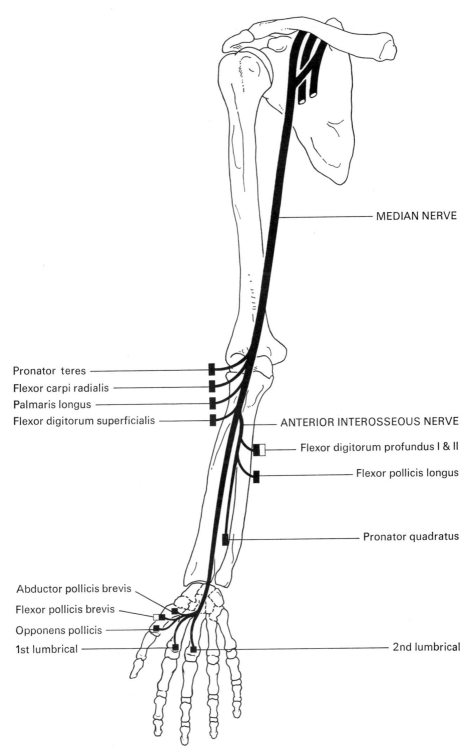

MEDIAN NERVE

Pronator teres

Flexor carpi radialis

Palmaris longus

Flexor digitorum superficialis

ANTERIOR INTEROSSEOUS NERVE

Flexor digitorum profundus I & II

Flexor pollicis longus

Pronator quadratus

Abductor pollicis brevis

Flexor pollicis brevis

Opponens pollicis

1st lumbrical

2nd lumbrical

Fig. 27 Diagram of the median nerve and the muscles which it supplies.
(Modified from Pitres and Testut). Note: the white rectangle signifies that the muscle indicated
receives a part of its nerve supply from another peripheral nerve (**cf** *Figs. 36, 45* and *46*).

25

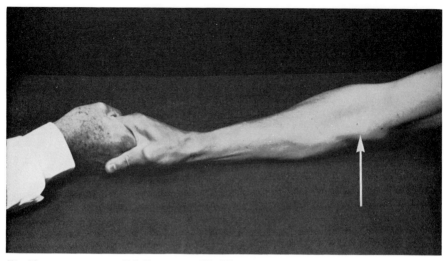

Fig. 28 PRONATOR TERES (Median nerve; C6, C7)
The patient is pronating the forearm against resistance. *Arrow:* the muscle belly can be felt and sometimes seen.

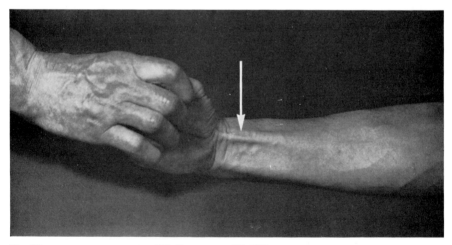

Fig. 29 FLEXOR CARPI RADIALIS (Median nerve; C6, C7)
The patient is flexing and abducting the hand at the wrist against resistance. *Arrow:* the tendon can be seen and felt.

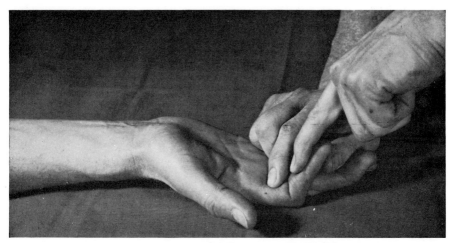

Fig. 30 FLEXOR DIGITORUM SUPERFICIALIS (Median nerve; C7, **C8**, T1)
The patient is flexing the finger at the proximal interphalangeal joint against resistance with the proximal phalanx fixed. This test does not eliminate the possibility of flexion at the proximal interphalangeal joint being produced by flexor digitorum profundus.

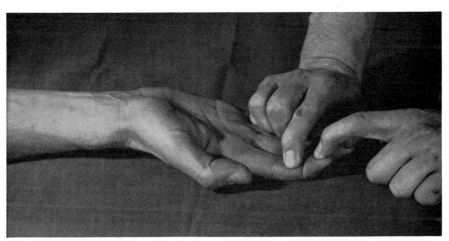

Fig. 31 FLEXOR DIGITORUM PROFUNDUS I AND II (Anterior interosseous nerve; C7, **C8**)
The patient is flexing the distal phalanx of the index finger against resistance with the middle phalanx fixed.

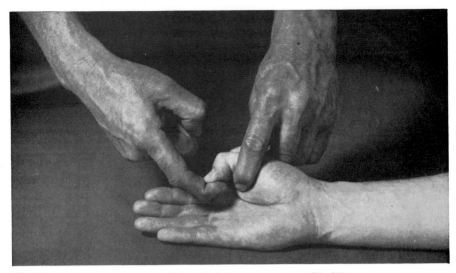

Fig. 32 FLEXOR POLLICIS LONGUS (Anterior interosseous nerve; C7, **C8**)
The patient is flexing the distal phalanx of the thumb against resistance while the proximal phalanx is fixed.

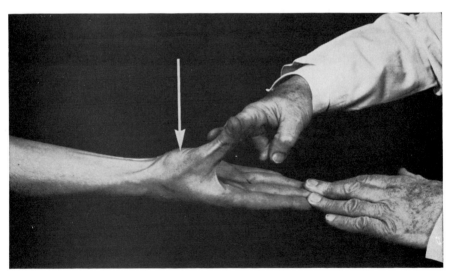

Fig. 33 ABDUCTOR POLLICIS BREVIS (Median nerve; C8, **T1**)
The patient is abducting the thumb at right angles to the palm against resistance.

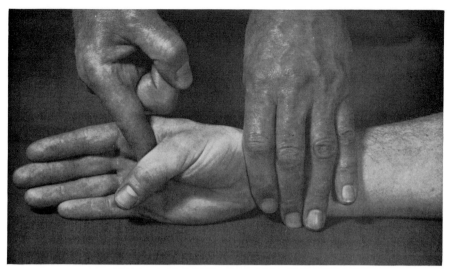

Fig. 34 OPPONENS POLLICIS (Median nerve; C8, **T1**)
The patient is touching the base of the little finger with the thumb against resistance.

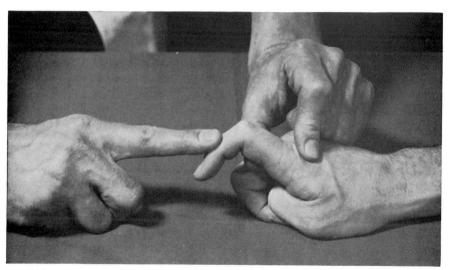

Fig. 35 1st LUMBRICAL-INTEROSSEOUS MUSCLE (Median and ulnar nerves: C8, **T1**)
The patient is extending the finger at the proximal interphalangeal joint against resistance with the metacarpophalangeal joint hyperextended and fixed.

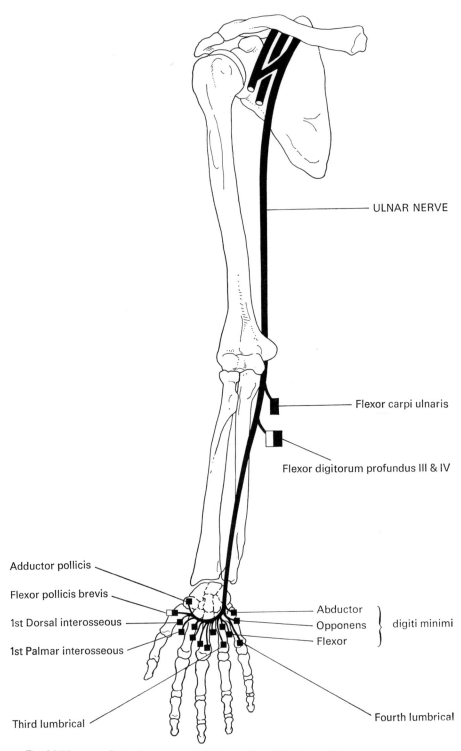

ULNAR NERVE

Flexor carpi ulnaris

Flexor digitorum profundus III & IV

Adductor pollicis

Flexor pollicis brevis

1st Dorsal interosseous

1st Palmar interosseous

Abductor

Opponens } digiti minimi

Flexor

Third lumbrical

Fourth lumbrical

Fig. 36 Diagram of the ulnar nerve and the muscles which it supplies. (Modified from Pitres and Testut)

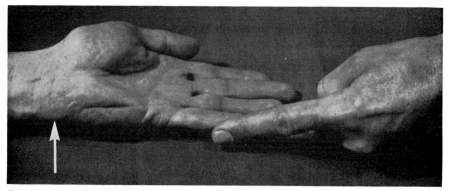

Fig. 37 FLEXOR CARPI ULNARIS (Ulnar nerve; C7, **C8**, T1)
The patient is abducting the little finger against resistance. The tendon of flexor carpi ulnaris can be seen and felt (arrow) as the muscle comes into action to fix the pisiform bone from which abductor digiti minimi arises. If flexor carpi ulnaris is intact, the tendon is seen even when abductor digiti minimi is paralyzed. (see also Fig. 38).

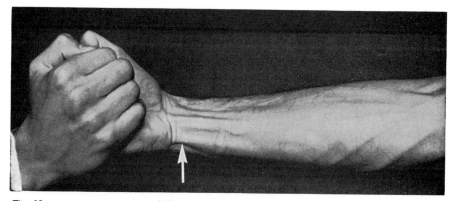

Fig. 38 FLEXOR CARPI ULNARIS (Ulnar nerve; C7, **C8**, T1)
The patient is flexing and adducting the hand at the wrist against resistance. *Arrow:* the tendon can be seen and felt.

31

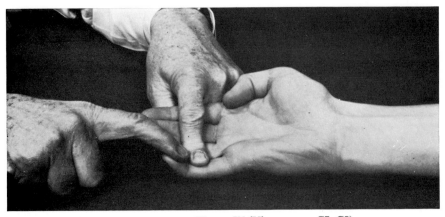

Fig. 39 FLEXOR DIGITORUM PROFUNDUS III AND IV (Ulnar nerve: C7, **C8**)
The patient is flexing the distal interphalangeal joint against resistance while the middle phalanx is fixed.

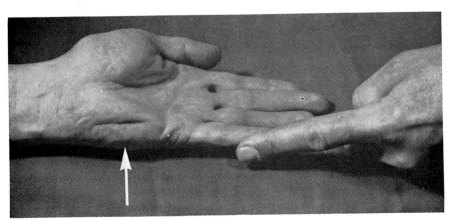

Fig. 40 ABDUCTOR DIGITI MINIMI (Ulnar nerve; C8, **T1**)
The back of the hand and fingers are flat upon the table. The patient is abducting the little finger against resistance. *Arrow:* the muscle belly can be felt and seen.

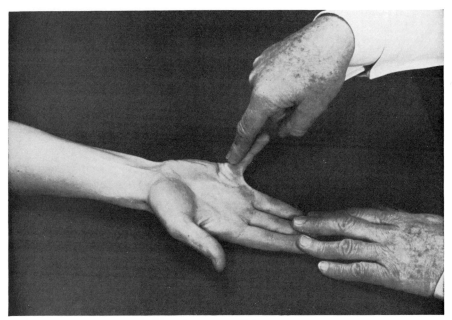

Fig. 41 FLEXOR DIGITI MINIMI (Ulnar nerve; C8, **T1**)
The patient is flexing the little finger at the metacarpophalangeal joint against resistance with the interphalangeal joints held extended.

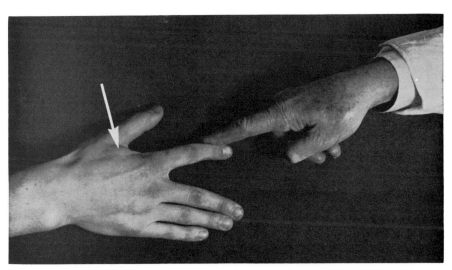

Fig. 42 FIRST DORSAL INTEROSSEOUS MUSCLE (Ulnar nerve; C8, **T1**)
The palm and fingers are flat upon a table. The patient is abducting the index finger against resistance. *Arrow:* the muscle belly can be felt and usually seen.

33

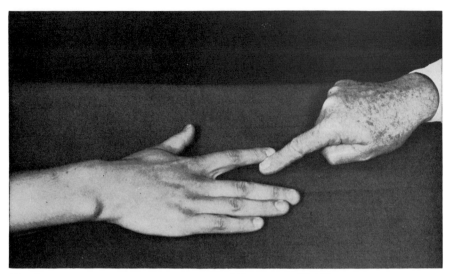

Fig. 43 SECOND PALMAR INTEROSSEOUS MUSCLE (Ulnar nerve; C8, **T1**)
The palm and fingers are flat upon a table. The patient is adducting the index finger against resistance.

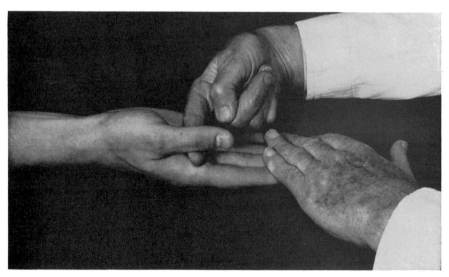

Fig. 44 ADDUCTOR POLLICIS (Ulnar nerve; C8, **T1**)
The patient is adducting the thumb at right angles to the palm against the resistance of the examiner's finger.

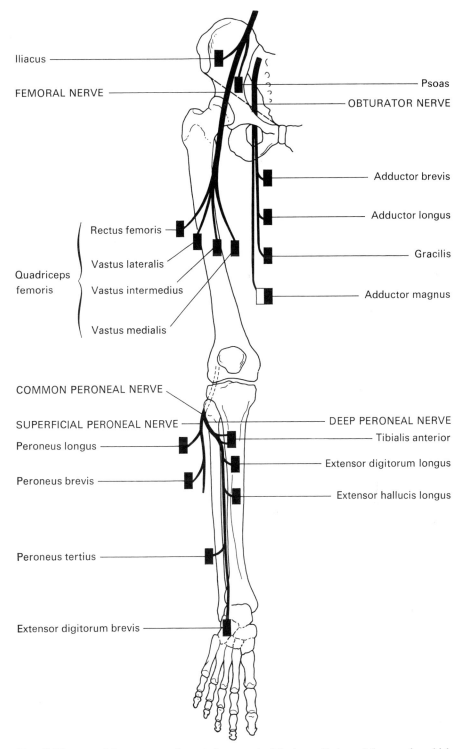

Iliacus

FEMORAL NERVE

Psoas

OBTURATOR NERVE

Adductor brevis

Adductor longus

Rectus femoris

Gracilis

Vastus lateralis

Quadriceps
femoris

Vastus intermedius

Adductor magnus

Vastus medialis

COMMON PERONEAL NERVE

SUPERFICIAL PERONEAL NERVE

DEEP PERONEAL NERVE

Tibialis anterior

Peroneus longus

Extensor digitorum longus

Peroneus brevis

Extensor hallucis longus

Peroneus tertius

Extensor digitorum brevis

Fig. 45 Diagram of the nerves on the anterior aspect of the lower limb, and the muscles which they supply. (Modified from Pitres and Testut)

35

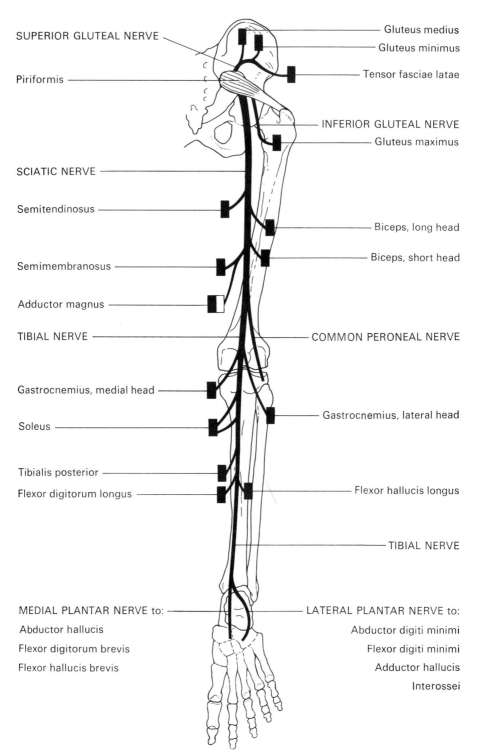

SUPERIOR GLUTEAL NERVE — Gluteus medius
— Gluteus minimus
Piriformis — — Tensor fasciae latae

INFERIOR GLUTEAL NERVE
— Gluteus maximus

SCIATIC NERVE —

Semitendinosus — — Biceps, long head

— Biceps, short head
Semimembranosus —

Adductor magnus —

TIBIAL NERVE — — COMMON PERONEAL NERVE

Gastrocnemius, medial head —

— Gastrocnemius, lateral head
Soleus —

Tibialis posterior —

Flexor digitorum longus — — Flexor hallucis longus

— TIBIAL NERVE

MEDIAL PLANTAR NERVE to: — — LATERAL PLANTAR NERVE to:
Abductor hallucis   Abductor digiti minimi
Flexor digitorum brevis   Flexor digiti minimi
Flexor hallucis brevis   Adductor hallucis
                                     Interossei

Fig. 46 Diagram of the nerves on the posterior aspect of the lower limb, and the muscles which they supply. (Modified from Pitres and Testut)

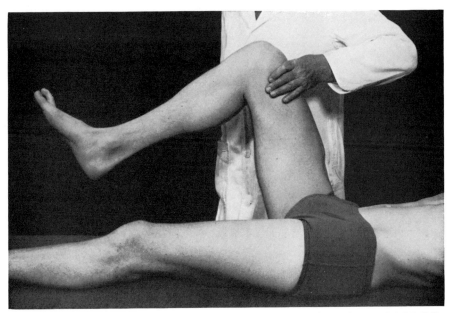

Fig. 47 ILIOPSOAS (Branches from L1, 2 and 3 spinal nerves and femoral nerve; **L1, L2,** L3)
The patient is flexing the thigh against resistance with the leg flexed at the knee and hip.

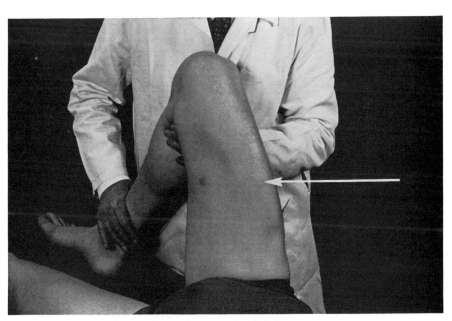

Fig. 48 QUADRICEPS FEMORIS (Femoral nerve; L2, **L3, L4**)
The patient is extending the leg against resistance with the limb flexed at the hip and knee. To detect slight weakness, the leg should be fully flexed at the knee. *Arrow:* the muscle belly of rectus femoris can be seen and felt.

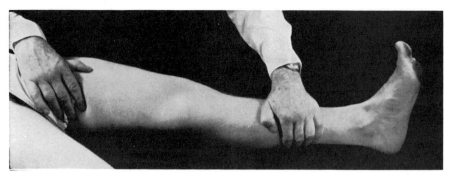

Fig. 49 ADDUCTORS (Obturator nerve; **L2, L3,** L4)
The patient lies on his back with the leg extended at the knee, and is adducting the limb against resistance. The muscle bellies can be felt.

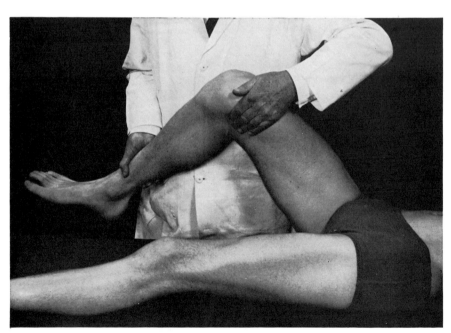

Fig. 50 GLUTEUS MEDIUS AND MINIMUS (Superior gluteal nerve; **L4, L5,** S1)
The patient lies on his back and is internally rotating the thigh against resistance with the limb flexed at the hip and knee.

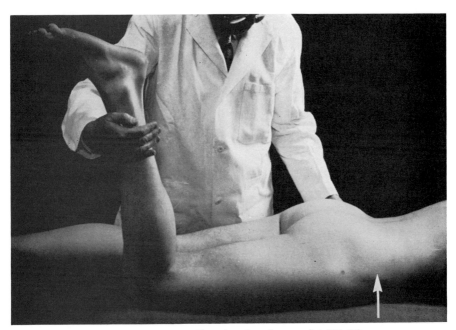

Fig. 51 GLUTEUS MEDIUS AND MINIMUS (Superior gluteal nerve; **L4, L5,** S1)
(An alternative method to that illustrated in Fig. 50). The patient lies on his face with the leg flexed at the knee to a right angle and is internally rotating the limb against resistance. *Arrow:* the muscle bellies can be felt and sometimes seen.

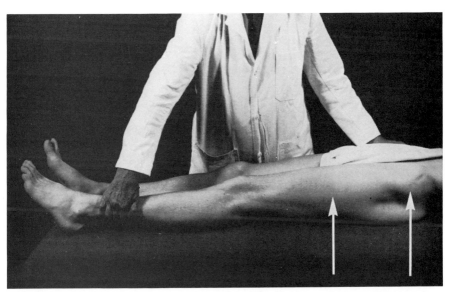

Fig. 52 GLUTEUS MEDIUS AND MINIMUS AND TENSOR FASCIAE LATAE (Superior gluteal nerve; **L4, L5,** S1)
The patient lies on his back with the leg extended and is abducting the limb against resistance. *Arrows:* the muscle bellies can be felt and sometimes seen.

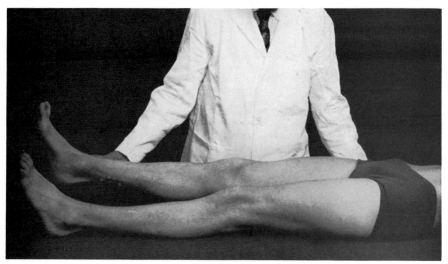

Fig. 53 GLUTEUS MAXIMUS (Inferior gluteal nerve; **L5, S1,** S2)
The patient lies on his back with the leg extended at the knee and is extending the limb at the
hip against resistance. The examiner's left hand is feeling the muscle.

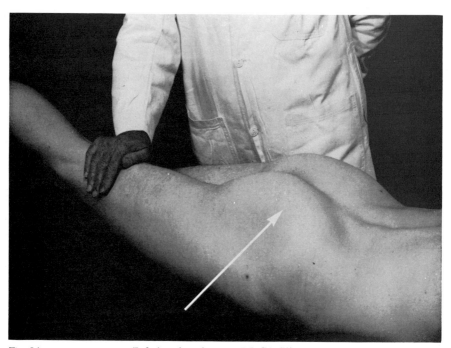

Fig. 54 GLUTEUS MAXIMUS (Inferior gluteal nerve; **L5, S1,** S2)
The patient lies on his face and is elevating the leg against resistance. *Arrow:* the muscle belly
can be felt and often seen.

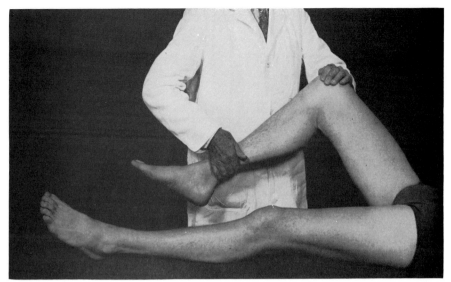

Fig. 55 HAMSTRING MUSCLES (Sciatic nerve. Semitendinosus, semimembranosus and biceps; L5, **S1, S2**)
The patient lies on his back with the limb flexed at the hip and knee and is flexing the leg at the knee against resistance.

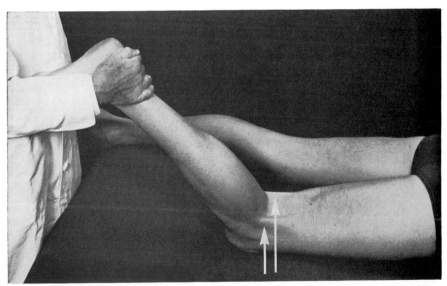

Fig. 56 HAMSTRING MUSCLES (Sciatic nerve. Semitendinosus, semimembranosus and biceps; L5, **S1.** S2)
The patient lies on his face and is flexing the leg at the knee against resistance. *Arrows:* the tendons of the biceps (laterally) and semitendinosus (medially) can be felt and usually seen.

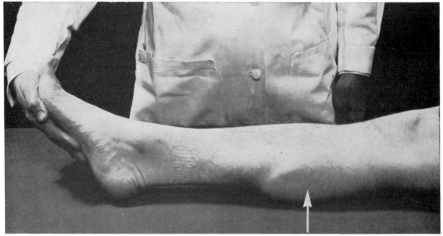

Fig. 57 GASTROCNEMIUS (Tibial nerve; S1, S2)
The patient lies on his back with the leg extended and is plantar-flexing the foot against resist-ance. *Arrow:* the muscle bellies can be seen and felt. To detect slight weakness, the patient should be asked to stand on one foot, raise the heel from the ground and maintain this position.

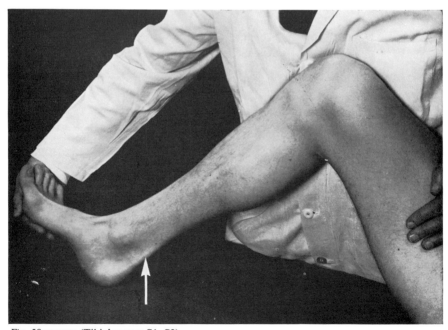

Fig. 58 SOLEUS (Tibial nerve; S1, S2)
The patient lies on his back with the limb flexed at the hip and knee and is plantar-flexing the foot against resistance. The muscle belly can be felt and sometimes seen. *Arrow:* the Achilles tendon.

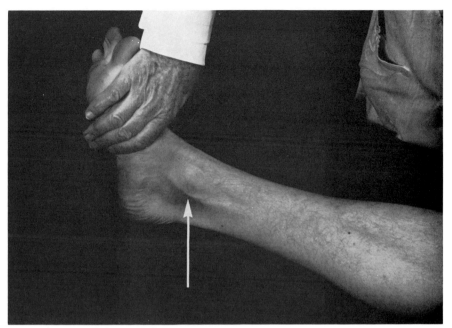

Fig. 59 TIBIALIS POSTERIOR (Tibial nerve; L4, L5)
The patient is inverting the foot against resistance. *Arrow:* the tendon can be seen and felt.

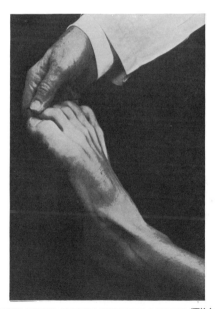

Fig. 60 FLEXOR DIGITORUM LONGUS, FLEXOR HALLUCIS LONGUS (Tibial nerve; L5, **S1, S2**)
The patient is flexing the toes against resistance.

43

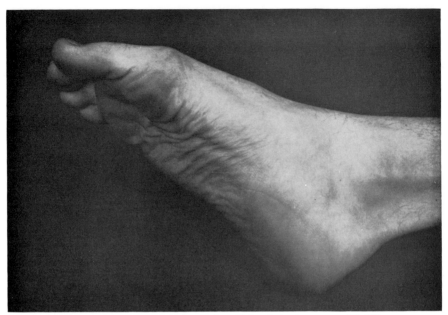

Fig. 61 SMALL MUSCLES OF THE FOOT (medial and lateral plantar nerves; S1, S2)
The patient is cupping the sole of the foot; the small muscles can be felt and sometimes seen.

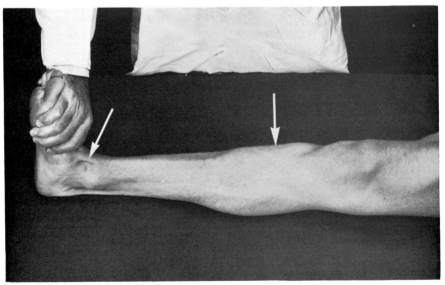

Fig. 62 TIBIALIS ANTERIOR (Deep peroneal nerve; L4, L5)
The patient is dorsiflexing the foot against resistance. *Arrows:* the muscle belly and its tendon can be seen and felt.

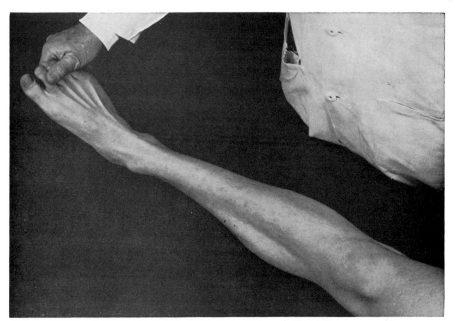

Fig. 63 EXTENSOR DIGITORUM LONGUS (Deep peroneal nerve; **L5, S1**)
The patient is dorsiflexing the toes against resistance. The tendons passing to the lateral four toes can be seen and felt.

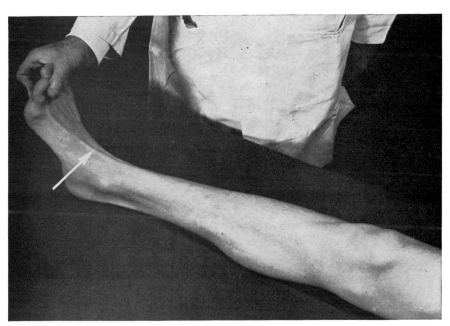

Fig. 64 EXTENSOR HALLUCIS LONGUS (Deep peroneal nerve; **L5, S1**)
The patient is dorsiflexing the distal phalanx of the big toe against resistance. *Arrow:* the tendon can be seen and felt.

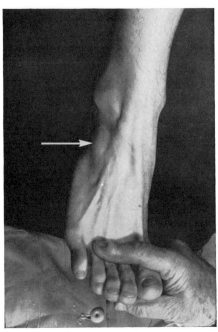

Fig. 65 EXTENSOR DIGITORUM BREVIS (Deep peroneal nerve; L5, S1)
The patient is dorsiflexing the proximal phalanges of the toes against resistance. *Arrow:* the muscle belly can be felt and sometimes seen.

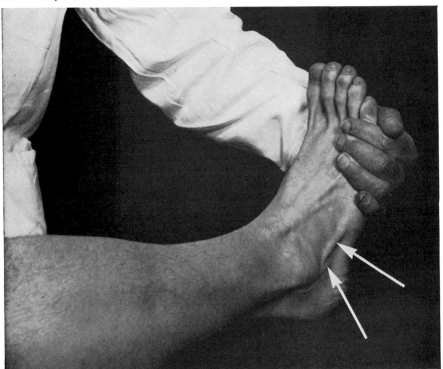

Fig. 66 PERONEUS LONGUS AND BREVIS (Superficial peroneal nerve; L5, S1)
The patient is everting the foot against resistance. *Upper arrow:* the tendon of peroneus brevis. *Lower arrow:* the tendon of peroneus longus.

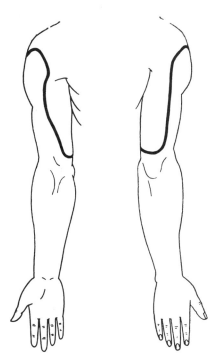

Fig. 67 The approximate area within which sensory changes may be found in complete lesions of the brachial plexus (C5, C6, C7, C8, T1).

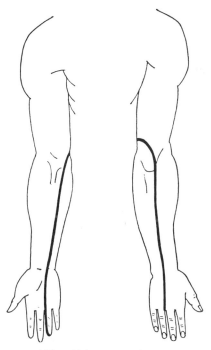

Fig. 68 The approximate area within which sensory changes may be found in lesions of the lower roots (C8, T1) of the brachial plexus.

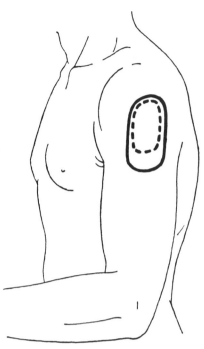

Fig. 69 The approximate area within which sensory changes may be found in lesions of the axillary nerve. Light touch, continuous line; pin-prick, dotted line.

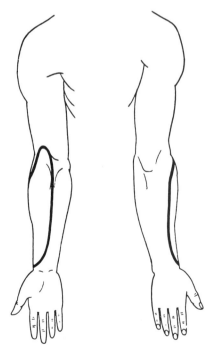

Fig. 70 The approximate area within which sensory changes may be found in lesions of the lateral cutaneous nerve of the forearm (the terminal branch of the musculocutaneous nerve).

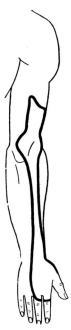

Fig. 71 The approximate area within which sensory changes may be found in high lesions of the radial nerve (above the origin of the posterior cutaneous nerves of the arm and forearm). The average area is usually considerably smaller, and absence of sensory changes has been recorded.

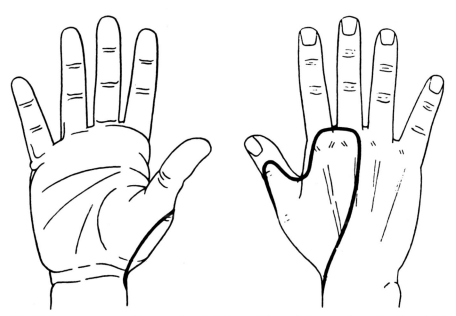

Fig. 72 An average area of sensory loss in lesions of the radial nerve above the elbow joint and below the origin of the posterior cutaneous nerve of the forearm.

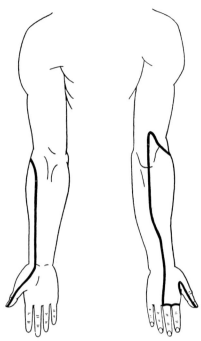

Fig. 73 The approximate area within which sensory changes may be found in combined lesions of the radial nerve (below the posterior cutaneous nerve of the arm) and musculocutaneous nerve.

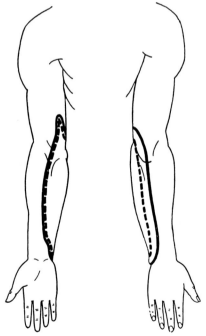

Fig. 74 The approximate area within which sensory changes may be found in lesions of the medial cutaneous nerve of the forearm. Light touch, continuous line; pin-prick, dotted line.

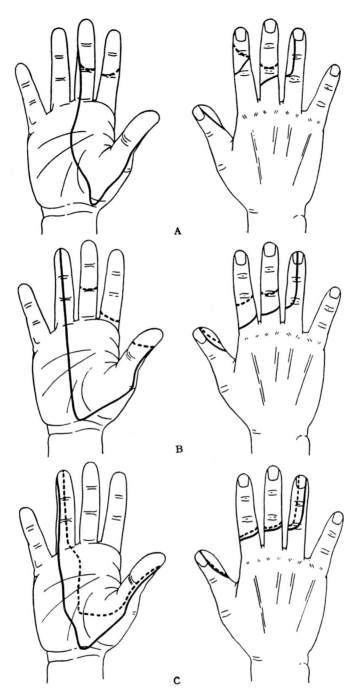

Fig. 75 (A, B and C). The approximate areas within which sensory changes may be found in lesions of the median nerve. A=small area, B=average area, and C=large area. Light touch, continuous line; pin-prick, dotted line. Immediately after complete division of the median nerve, the insensitive area on the palm of the hand may be somewhat larger than is shown. (Modified from Head and Sherren (1905) *Brain*, **28**, 116)

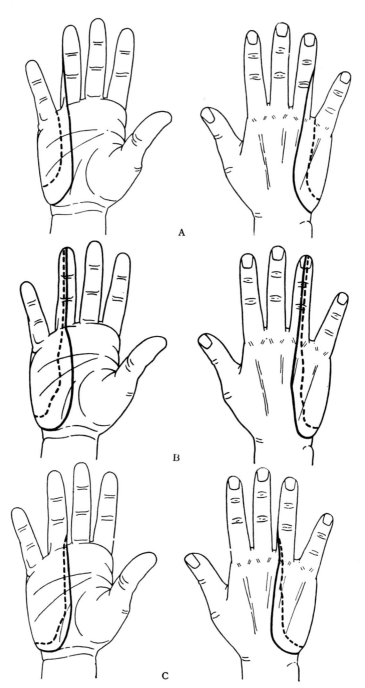

Fig. 76 (A, B and C). The approximate areas within which sensory changes may be found in lesions of the ulnar nerve. A=small area, B=average area, and C=large area. Light touch, continuous line; pin-prick, dotted line. Immediately after complete division of the ulnar nerve, the insensitive area on the palm of the hand may be somewhat larger than is shown. (Modified from Head and Sherren)

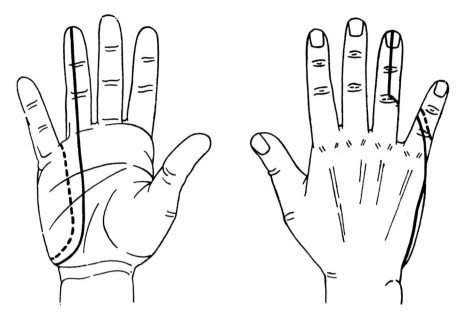

Fig. 77 The approximate area within which sensory changes may be found in lesions of the ulnar nerve below the origin of its dorsal branch. Light touch, continuous line; pin-prick, dotted line. (Modified from Head and Sherren)

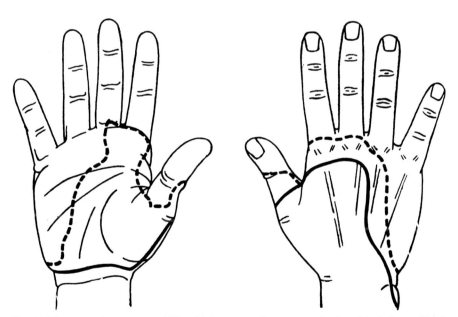

Fig. 78 The approximate area within which sensory changes may be found in lesions of both median and ulnar nerves. Light touch, continuous line; pin-prick, dotted line. (Modified from M.R.C. Special Reports No. 54, 1920, H.M.S.O., London)

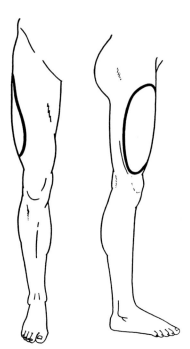

Fig. 79 The approximate area within which sensory changes may be found in lesions of the lateral cutaneous nerve of the thigh.

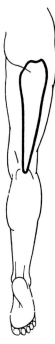

Fig. 80 The approximate area within which sensory changes may be found in lesions of the posterior cutaneous nerve of the thigh.

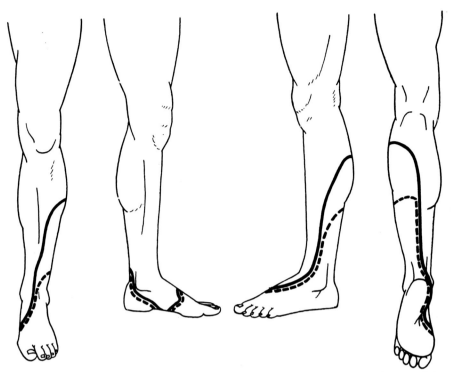

Fig. 81 The approximate area within which sensory changes may be found in lesions of the trunk of the sciatic nerve. Light touch, continuous line; pin-prick, dotted line. (Modified from M.R.C. Special Report No. 54, 1920)

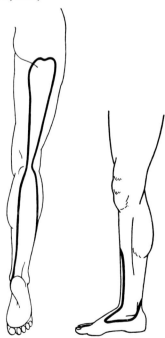

Fig. 82 The approximate area within which sensory changes may be found in lesions of both the sciatic and the posterior cutaneous nerve of the thigh.

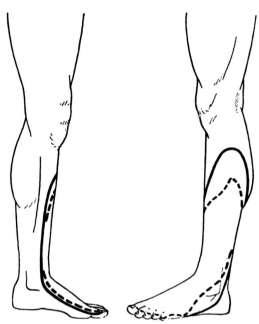

Fig. 83 The approximate area within which sensory changes may be found in lesions of the common peroneal nerve above the origin of the superficial peroneal nerve. Light touch, continuous line; pin-prick, dotted line. (Modified from M.R.C. Special Report No. 54, 1920)

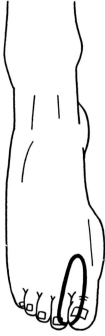

Fig. 84 The approximate area within which sensory changes may be found in lesions of the deep peroneal nerve.

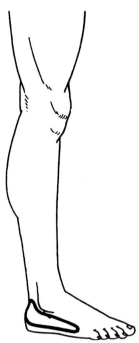

Fig. 85 The approximate area within which sensory changes may be found in lesions of the sural nerve.

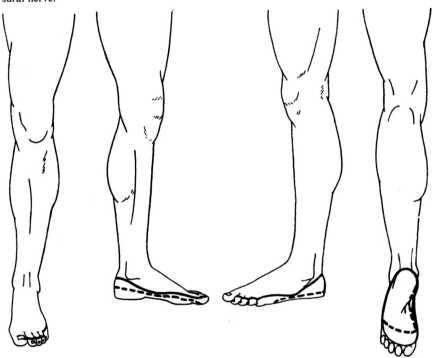

Fig. 86 The approximate area within which sensory changes may be found in lesions of the tibial nerve. Light touch, continuous line; pin-prick, dotted line. (Modified from M.R.C. Special Report No. 54, 1920)

Figs. 87–90 show the approximate cutaneous areas supplied by each spinal root (after Foerster (1933), *Brain*, **56**, 1.). There is considerable variation and overlap between dermatomes so that an isolated root lesion results in a much smaller area of sensory impairment than is indicated in these diagrams.

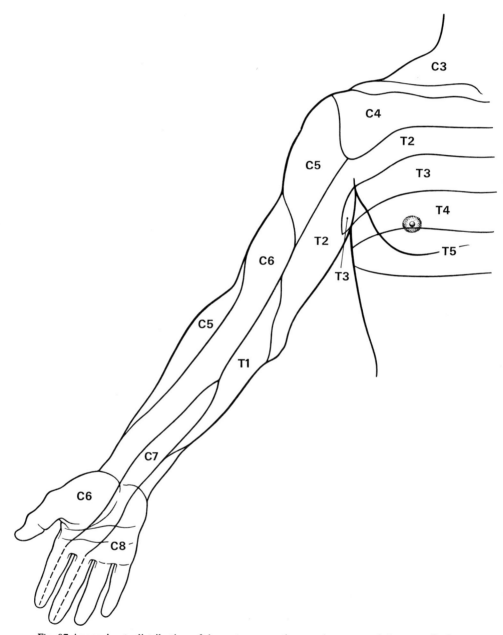

Fig. 87 Approximate distribution of dermatomes on the anterior aspect of the upper limb.

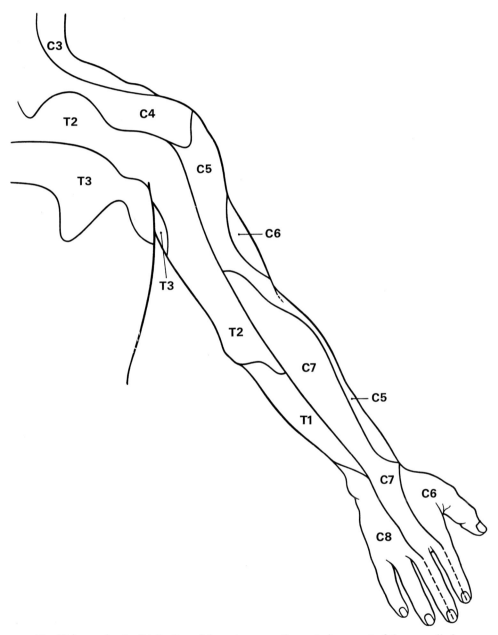

Fig. 88 Approximate distribution of dermatomes on the posterior aspect of the upper limb.

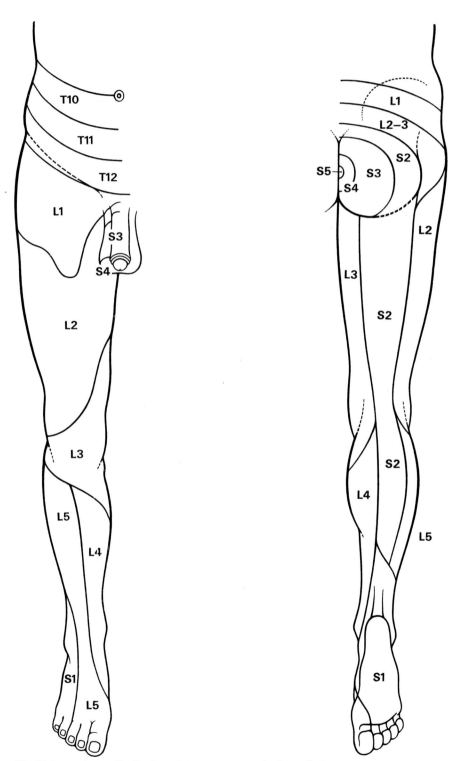

Fig. 89 Approximate distribution of dermatomes on the lower limb.

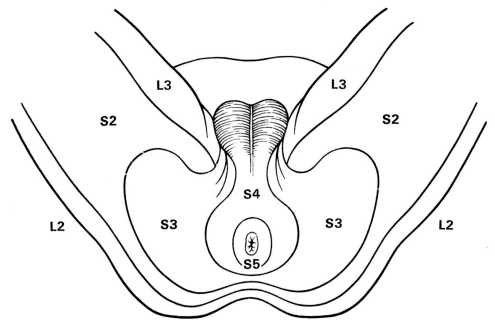

Fig. 90 Approximate distribution of dermatomes on the perineum.

Nerve and main root supply of muscles

(The list given below does not include all the muscles innervated by these nerves, but only those more commonly tested, either clinically or electrically, and shows the order of innervation.)

UPPER LIMB	Spinal Roots
Spinal Accessory Nerve	
Trapezius	C3, C4
Brachial Plexus	
Rhomboids	C4, C5
Serratus anterior	C5, C6, C7
Pectoralis major	
Clavicular	**C5**, C6
Sternal	C6, **C7**, C8
Supraspinatus	**C5**, C6
Infraspinatus	**C5**, C6
Latissimus dorsi	C6, **C7**, C8
Teres major	C5, 6, 7
Axillary Nerve	
Deltoid	**C5**, C6
Musculocutaneous Nerve	
Biceps	C5, C6
Brachialis	C5, C6
Radial Nerve	
Triceps { Long head / Lateral head / Medial head }	C6, **C7**, C8
Brachioradialis	C5, **C6**
Extensor carpi radialis longus	C5, **C6**
Posterior Interosseous Nerve	
Supinator	C6, C7
Extensor carpi ulnaris	**C7**, C8
Extensor digitorum	**C7**, C8
Abductor pollicis longus	**C7**, C8
Extensor pollicis longus	**C7**, C8
Extensor pollicis brevis	**C7**, C8
Extensor indicis	**C7**, C8
Median Nerve	
Pronator teres	C6, C7
Flexor carpi radialis,	C6, C7
Flexor digitorum superficialis	C7, **C8**, T1
Abductor pollicis brevis	C8, **T1**
Flexor pollicis brevis*	C8, **T1**
Opponens pollicis	C8, **T1**
Lumbricals I & II	C8, **T1**
Anterior Interosseous Nerve	
Flexor digitorum profundus I & II	C7, **C8**
Flexor pollicis longus	C7, **C8**
Ulnar Nerve	
Flexor carpi ulnaris	C7, **C8**, T1
Flexor digitorum profundus III & IV	C7, **C8**
Hypothenar muscles	C8, **T1**
Adductor pollicis	C8, **T1**
Flexis pollicis brevis	C8, **T1**
Palmar interossei	C8, **T1**
Dorsal interossei	C8, **T1**
Lumbricals III & IV	C8, **T1**

LOWER LIMB	Spinal Roots
Femoral Nerve	
Iliopsoas	**L1, L2**, L3
Rectus femoris ⎫	
Vastus lateralis ⎬ Quadriceps	
Vastus intermedius ⎪ femoris	**L2, L3, L4**
Vastus medialis ⎭	
Obturator Nerve	
Adductor longus ⎱	
Adductor magnus ⎰	**L2, L3**, L4
Superior Gluteal Nerve ⎫	
Gluteus medius and minimus ⎬	**L4, L5**, S1
Tensor fasciae latae ⎭	
Inferior Gluteal Nerve	
Gluteus maximus	**L5, S1**, S2
Sciatic and Tibial Nerves	
Semitendinosus	L5, **S1**, S2
Biceps	L5, **S1**, S2
Semimembranosus	L5, **S1**, S2
Gastrocnemius and soleus	S1, S2
Tibialis posterior	L4, L5
Flexor digitorum longus	L5, **S1, S2**
Flexor hallucis longus	L5, **S1, S2**
Abductor hallucis ⎱ Small muscles	S1, S2
Abductor digiti minimi ⎬ of foot	
Interossei ⎰	
Sciatic and Common Peroneal Nerves	
Tibialis anterior	**L4**, L5
Extensor digitorum longus	**L5**, S1
Extensor hallucis longus	**L5**, S1
Extensor digitorum brevis	L5, S1
Peroneus longus	L5, S1
Peroneus brevis	L5, S1

*Flexor pollicis brevis is often supplied wholly or partially by the ulnar nerve.

Printed in the United States of America
for Pendragon House, Inc.,
by the George Banta Co., Inc., of
Menasha, Wisconsin.